NAUSEA

BRIEFLY EXPLORING THE WORLD OF

NAUSEA

DR. A. RAMOS

Contents

INTRODUCTION

A complex and unpleasant feeling, nausea is frequently accompanied by the desire to throw up. It is merely a symptom that may be brought on by a number of underlying conditions rather than a particular disease. There are two types of nausea: acute, which lasts briefly, and chronic, which lasts for a longer time. Although it is frequently associated with gastrointestinal problems, such infections or motion sickness, it can also be a sign of a number of other illnesses, pregnancy, or pharmaceutical side effects.

Anxiety is a feeling that is influenced by both psychological and physiological elements. Nausea is the body's natural reaction to discomfort or possible harm. It works as a deterrent to prevent people from ingesting dangerous drugs.

Other symptoms that may accompany nausea include perspiration, lightheadedness, increased salivation, and overall discomfort. There are many different reasons why people get nauseated, from hormone fluctuations and psychological factors to infections and digestive problems.

The goal of managing nausea is to treat its underlying cause. Depending on the individual case, this may entail medication, dietary adjustments, lifestyle changes, or other interventions. It is best to seek medical attention for a comprehensive evaluation and suitable direction if the condition is severe or persistent.

Though nausea is not an illness in and of itself, it can have a serious negative effect on a person's health and quality of life. For effective therapy and relief from nausea, it is essential to identify and treat the underlying cause of the condition.

CHAPTER ONE

The Physiology and Anatomy of Nausea

Many physiological systems in the body are involved in the complicated physiological response known as nausea, and both physical and psychological variables can affect how nausea feels. Gaining knowledge about the morphology and physiology of nausea will help you better understand the complex processes that lead to this feeling.

1. The central nervous system (CNS) and the brain:

The feeling of nausea is mostly mediated by the brain. Situated in the medulla oblongata, the vomiting center is an essential region that receives signals from several regions of the body. It combines data from higher brain areas, the vestibular system in the inner ear, and the gastrointestinal tract.

2. The digestive tract

Nausea is closely associated with the digestive system. Transmission of signals to the vomiting center might occur from irritation or inflammation of the intestines, stomach lining, or other digestive organs. Nausea can be brought on by illnesses such intestinal obstructions, gastritis, or gastroenteritis.

3. Vestibular System:

The vestibular system of the inner ear, which is in charge of balance and spatial orientation, plays a role in both equilibrium and motion perception. Nausea can result from disturbances in this system, such as those caused by inner ear problems or motion sickness.

4. Trigger Zone for Chemoreceptors (CTZ):

The brain's postrema region contains the chemoreceptor trigger zone, which is sensitive to a variety of bloodstream substances. Toxins, drugs, or changes in metabolism can all stimulate it and cause nausea.

5. System Nervous Autonomic:

Bodily functions are regulated by the sympathetic and parasympathetic branches of the autonomic nervous system. Sweating and an elevated heart rate are two symptoms that might result from the sympathetic nervous system being activated, which is linked to nausea.

6. Hormonal Elements:

Nausea may be exacerbated by hormonal changes, especially during pregnancy, menstruation, or certain medical diseases. Hormones including human chorionic gonadotropin (hCG) contribute to nausea associated with pregnancy.

7. Emotional and Psychological Aspects:

Feelings and psychological elements, such as tension, worry, or exposure to stressful events, might affect how sick one feels. The vomiting center interacts with the limbic system of the brain, which is involved with emotions and memory.

8. Perceptual Data:

Nausea can result from sensory input coming from a variety of receptors, including taste and smell receptors. Unpleasant tastes, smells, or textures could cause the feeling.

9. Blood Flow:

Nausea can be exacerbated by blood circulation abnormalities, such as low blood sugar or decreased blood supply to the brain.

Healthcare providers can more effectively diagnose and treat the underlying causes of nausea when they are aware of how these systems are interrelated. Managing underlying medical issues, treating psychological or lifestyle variables that contribute to nausea, and symptom relief are among possible treatment approaches.

Typical Reasons for Nausea

Numerous things can cause nausea, so figuring out what's causing it is crucial to managing it effectively. Some typical causes of nausea are as follows:

Digestive Disorders:

Gastritis: Inflammation brought on by bacterial or viral infections of the stomach and intestines.

Gastritis: Inflammation of the lining of the stomach, frequently brought on by drugs, alcohol, or infections.

Peptic Ulcers: Wounds that appear on the upper small intestine or stomach lining.

infections

Nausea is a symptom of several illnesses, including urinary tract infections, norovirus, and influenza (flu).

Motion Vertigo:

vestibular disruption, which frequently occurs during flights, boat voyages, and automobile rides.

Headaches:

severe headaches that are frequently accompanied by light and sound sensitivities and nausea.

Drugs:

Nausea is a side effect of certain medications, such as opioid painkillers, chemotherapy treatments, and some antibiotics.

Being pregnant:

Early in a pregnancy, nausea and vomiting also referred to as morning sickness are typical.

Changes in Hormones:

Nausea may be exacerbated by hormonal changes that occur during menopause or the menstrual cycle.

Foodborne Illness:

eating tainted food, which causes gastrointestinal symptoms like nausea and vomiting.

GERD, or gastroesophageal reflux disease:

Prolonged acid reflux can irritate the esophagus, which can result in nausea.

Stress & Anxiety:

Nausea can be brought on by psychological variables as stress, worry, or emotional anguish.

Indulging in excess:

Eating a lot of food can cause the digestive system to become overwhelmed, which can cause nausea.

An appendix is:

Pain and nausea in the abdomen might result from appendix inflammation.

Pancreatitis:

Pancreatic inflammation, frequently accompanied by nausea and stomach pain.

Stones in the kidney:

Kidney stones can hurt and make you feel sick.

Chemotherapy:

Chemotherapy and other cancer treatments can cause nausea as a side effect.

Intoxication with alcohol:

Drinking too much alcohol can irritate the lining of the stomach, which can cause nausea and vomiting.

Specific Scents or Odors:

Some people get queasy when they smell something strong or unpleasant.

Dehydration:

Nausea may arise from conditions leading to dehydration or from inadequate fluid intake.

It's crucial to remember that every person reacts differently to triggers, so this list is not all-inclusive. A medical expert should be consulted if nausea is severe or persistent in order to identify the underlying cause and the best course of action.

Symptoms and Indications

Numerous indications and symptoms that add to the overall discomfort are frequently present with nausea. These can differ from person to person and could consist of:

Unease:

a generalized stomach ache or discomfort that is frequently referred to as uneasy.

Enhanced Appetiteness

oversimplification of salivation or a feeling of "watery mouth."

Perspiration:

increased sweating, particularly on the hands and forehead.

Feeling lightheaded:

a dizzy or lightheaded feeling that could be more intense when standing or moving.

Paleness:

skin pallor, occasionally paired with chilly sweats.

Breathing Quickly:

shallow or fast breathing, frequently brought on by discomfort or stress in the body.

Retching:

the uncontrollably rhythmic contraction of the vomiting-related muscles, even in the absence of vomiting.

Excessive salivation

excessive salivation, which makes swallowing necessary more often.

Heartburn:

a burning feeling in the chest that is frequently a sign of GERD, or acid reflux illness.

Uncomfortable Stomach:

Abdominal pain or discomfort that can range in intensity from minor to severe.

Weakness

a weak or lethargic feeling that could be brought on by the stress reaction.

Fear:

feelings of unease or fear, which can either cause or be brought on by nausea.

Elevated heart rate

an increased heart rate, linked to the body's reaction to discomfort or stress.

Diminished Appetite:

a decreased appetite or an allergy to food, frequently linked to nausea.

Smell Sensitivity:

increased sensitivity to fragrances, with some scents causing or aggravating nausea.

During Particular Activities:

motion sickness is a type of nausea brought on by specific activities, such reading while driving.

Throwing up:

There are situations when nausea turns into genuine vomiting, which causes the stomach contents to come out.

It's critical to remember that nausea is a symptom, not a particular illness.

CHAPTER TWO

Healthcare practitioners can identify possible underlying reasons and choose the best course of action for management and alleviation with the aid of the accompanying signs and symptoms. A healthcare professional should be consulted if nausea is severe or persistent in order to receive a thorough evaluation and customized treatment plan.

Diagnosis and Assessment

When diagnosing and treating nausea, medical professionals must do a thorough assessment in order to pinpoint the underlying cause and choose the best course of action. The following steps could be part of the process:

Health Background:

The patient's medical history, including the beginning and duration of the nausea, any accompanying symptoms, any known medical conditions, medications, recent travel, dietary practices, and exposure to any toxins, will be gathered by the healthcare professional.

Physical Assessment:

In order to evaluate vital signs, abdominal soreness, dehydration symptoms, and other pertinent physical findings, a comprehensive physical examination may be performed.

Evaluation of Drugs:

The patient's current medications will be reviewed by the healthcare professional because certain medications have a side effect of nausea or can exacerbate it.

Laboratory Examinations:

Blood tests can be performed to check for anomalies such as electrolyte imbalances, liver or renal function, infections, and other conditions.

Imaging Research:

Imaging tests like magnetic resonance imaging (MRI), computed tomography (CT) scans, or abdominal ultrasonography (US) may be suggested to view the organs and detect any anomalies, depending on the probable underlying reason.

Endoscopy:

The gastrointestinal system can be directly visualized with endoscopic procedures like esophagogastroduodenoscopy (EGD) or colonoscopy, which can help detect problems including inflammation, ulcers, or structural anomalies.

Pregnancy Examination:

Given that nausea is frequently a sign of early pregnancy in people of reproductive age, a pregnancy test may be performed to either confirm or rule out pregnancy.

Assessment of Psychological Elements:

When psychological issues are suspected of playing a role in nausea, a mental health assessment could be advised to rule out illnesses like depression or anxiety.

Evaluation of Eating Behaviors:

To look for links between dietary variables and nausea, an assessment of dietary practices and potential foodborne infections may be undertaken.

Evaluation of Motion Sickness:

If a patient is suffering from motion sickness-related nausea, the doctor could ask about particular travel circumstances or activities that set off symptoms.

Assessment of Correlated Symptoms:

To reduce the number of possible reasons, the existence of concomitant symptoms like fever, stomach pain, bowel habit changes, or neurological symptoms will be taken into account.

The diagnosis procedure is customized based on the unique symptoms and medical background of the patient. Accurate diagnosis depends on the patient and the healthcare professional working together. A focused treatment strategy can be put into place to successfully address the nausea and its accompanying symptoms after the underlying cause has been found. Referrals to obstetricians, neurologists, or gastroenterologists for additional assessment and care may be taken into consideration if necessary.

The goal of treating nausea is to alleviate the underlying cause of the condition as well as the nausea itself. Treatment strategies can change depending on the particular cause and patient conditions. Here are some typical methods for treating nausea:

Handling the Root Causes:

For nausea to be effectively treated, the underlying cause must be found and addressed. This could entail managing chronic illnesses, treating infections, modifying medication, or taking care of other underlying causes.

Drugs:

Antiemetic drugs are frequently administered to treat nausea and stop vomiting. These drugs could consist of:

Antihistamines: Often used to treat motion sickness, such as dimenhydrinate or meclizine.

Metoclopramide and prochlorperazine are examples of dopamine receptor antagonists that lessen nausea and vomiting.

Similar to ondansetron, serotonin receptor antagonists are frequently used to prevent and treat nausea brought on by chemotherapy or surgery.

Dietary Adjustments:

Depending on the underlying reason of the nausea, dietary modifications could be advised. This may entail eating bland foods, avoiding trigger foods, and drinking plenty of water.

Drinking plenty of water

Drinking enough water is crucial, particularly if dehydration is accompanied by nausea. It can be advised to take little sips of clear liquids or oral rehydration solutions.

Ginger:

Because of its antiemetic qualities, ginger may help lessen nausea. It can be eaten in many different ways, including in ginger tea or ginger candy. Before taking ginger supplements, people should consult their doctor, especially if they have certain medical concerns.

Acupressure:

Acupressure, especially bracelets or pressure on particular acupuncture points, helps some people who are feeling sick to their stomach. But the degree to which it works depends on the individual.

Psychological Assistance:

Counseling or stress-reduction methods may be helpful for nausea caused by psychological, anxiety, or stress-related issues.

Preventing Motion Sickness:

If you experience nausea when traveling, you may find it helpful to take preventive precautions including wearing motion sickness wristbands, taking breaks, and keeping your eyes on the horizon.

Methods Particular to Pregnancy:

It may be advised to make dietary adjustments, lifestyle adjustments, and, in certain situations, prescription medication, to treat morning sickness during pregnancy. A typical treatment for nausea associated with pregnancy is a combination of vitamin B6 and doxylamine.

Steer clear of trigger factors:

Managing nausea can be aided by recognizing and avoiding particular triggers, such as particular foods, fragrances, or activities.

It's critical that people with severe or chronic nausea speak with a healthcare professional for an in-depth assessment and individualized treatment plan. The underlying cause will determine the treatment plan, and good management depends on regular communication between the patient and medical staff.

Nutritional Aspects

Dietary factors are important in the management of nausea, particularly when it is linked to certain illnesses or triggers. Specific dietary adjustments can offer relief and help with symptoms. The following food recommendations will help you manage your nausea:

bland foods

Choose meals that are simple to digest and bland. The BRAT diet has toast, applesauce, bananas, rice, and plain crackers as examples. These foods are less prone to cause nausea and are easier on the stomach.

Little, Regular Meals:

Eat smaller, more frequent meals throughout the day as opposed to one big meal. This can lessen the chance of nausea by keeping the stomach from getting too full.

Do Not Inhale Strong Odors:

Strong smells can cause nausea or exacerbate it. Steer clear of cooking or being near strongly scented food, and opt for less aromatic foods that are cool or room temperature.

Ginger:

Because of its antiemetic qualities, ginger may help lessen nausea. Ginger tea, ginger candy, or ginger ale are some ways to include ginger in your diet. But before taking ginger supplements, especially if you have specific medical issues, speak with your doctor.

Transparent Liquids:

Drink clear liquids to stay hydrated, such as water, fruit juice that has been diluted, or clear broths. Staying hydrated is crucial since dehydration can make nausea worse.

Keeping Trigger Foods Away:

Recognize and stay away from particular meals and drinks that make you queasy. Caffeine, strong-flavored foods, greasy or fatty foods, and spicy or spicy foods are common triggers.

Cold Foods:

It could be easier to tolerate cold meals than heated ones. Think about eating cold foods or snacks, including smoothies, yogurt, or cold fruits.

Crystallized peppermint or ginger:

Some people get relief from nausea by sucking on peppermint or crystallized ginger candies. These may have a gentle, calming impact.

Rich in Protein Snacks:

Include high-protein snacks in your diet, like lean proteins, boiled eggs, or plain yogurt. Protein has the ability to increase feelings of fullness and normalize blood sugar levels.

Foods High in Acid:

Steer clear of extremely acidic foods and drinks since they may aggravate the lining of the stomach. Citrus fruits, tomatoes, and acidic juices are examples of this.

Easy Crackers or Dehydrated Toast:

Dry toast or plain crackers might be a good alternative for calming the stomach, especially if they are consumed gradually in little amounts.

Steer Clear of Too Sweet Foods:

While eating sweet foods can help some people feel better when they're sick, others might not be able to handle flavors that are too sweet. The key is moderation.

It's crucial to remember that different diets may be advised depending on the underlying reason of nausea. For a comprehensive assessment and individualized advice, it is recommended to speak with a healthcare professional if nausea is severe or continues. Additionally, for particular nutritional advice throughout pregnancy, pregnant women who are suffering morning sickness should speak with their healthcare professional.

Coping Mechanisms and Ways to Change Your Lifestyle

A combination of lifestyle changes and effective symptom management techniques are used to cope with nausea. The following coping mechanisms and way of life adjustments can help with nausea:

Relaxation and Rest:

Sufficient rest and relaxation can aid in reducing stress, which has been linked to nausea. Engage in relaxation exercises like yoga, meditation, or deep breathing.

Acupressure:

Take into consideration acupressure wristbands that are made to provide pressure to P6 or Nei-Kuan points, which are particular acupuncture sites. These bracelets help some people who are feeling sick to their stomach.

Supplements with ginger:

Consider taking ginger tablets or capsules after seeing a healthcare professional. They may help lessen nausea. Talking about dose and possible drug interactions is crucial, though.

Aromatherapy:

Using aromatherapy to relieve nausea, try using fragrances like ginger or peppermint. It can be beneficial to inhale these aromas or use essential oils in a diffuser.

Drinking plenty of water

Drink plenty of clear liquids to be well-hydrated throughout the day. It's important to keep your fluid balance because dehydration might make nausea worse.

Chilled Compress:

Relieving nausea and providing comfort can be achieved by placing a cold compress on the forehead or back of the neck.

Steer clear of triggers:

Recognize and stay away from things that make you feel queasy. This could include particular meals, powerful smells, or activities that exacerbate the symptoms.

Dietary Adjustments:

To manage nausea, adhere to dietary advice, such as choosing foods that are bland and readily absorbed. Think about eating smaller, more often meals instead of larger ones.

Orientation:

Try a variety of body positions to see which one feels most comfortable. For other people, sitting up straight or slightly reclining is a relief.

Techniques for Distraction:

Take part in activities that can divert your attention from nausea, like reading a book, watching a movie, or listening to relaxing music.

Consciously Consuming Food:

Eat with awareness by taking tiny nibbles and chewing your meal thoroughly. This can lessen the chance of feeling queasy and help avoid overindulging.

Coping Unique to Pregnancy:

Try having some plain toast or dry crackers before getting out of bed in the morning if you're pregnant and experiencing morning sickness. It might also be beneficial to have little, frequent snacks during the day.

Interaction with the Healthcare Provider:

Keep lines of communication open with your healthcare practitioner about your symptoms, triggers, and the efficacy of coping mechanisms. It can be advised to make therapeutic modifications or provide more assistance.

It's critical to keep in mind that different people may respond to coping mechanisms in different ways, and that what works for one person may not work for another. For a comprehensive assessment and individualized advice, it is recommended to speak with a healthcare professional if nausea is severe or continues. Additionally, for special advice during pregnancy, expectant mothers should speak with their healthcare professional.

Constant nausea can be unsettling and could be a sign of a serious medical condition that needs to be treated. While occasional and transient nausea is common and may not warrant medical attention, severe or chronic nausea, particularly when accompanied by specific warning signs, should be evaluated by a doctor. The following are some warning signs of chronic nausea that need to be addressed right away:

Unexpected Loss of Weight:

Sustaining nausea combined with inexplicable weight loss may be a sign of several underlying illnesses, such as cancer, metabolic problems, or gastrointestinal ailments.

CHAPTER THREE

Severe Pain in the Abdomen:

Severe abdominal discomfort coupled with nausea, especially if localized and ongoing, may indicate illnesses like pancreatitis, appendicitis, or intestinal blockage.

Blood in the Stool or Vomit:

Blood in the stool (melena) or vomit (hematemesis) indicates possible bleeding in the digestive tract. This needs to be treated medically right now.

Dehydration:

Extreme thirst, dark urine, infrequent urination, and dry mouth are all indicators of dehydration, which can lead to severe nausea or an underlying medical condition that has to be treated.

Extended Period:

If nausea doesn't go away after a long time, it can be a sign of a persistent illness that has to be looked into.

Symptoms related to the nervous system:

When neurological symptoms such a strong headache, blurred vision, or loss of coordination are present along with nausea, these could be signs of neurological diseases or migraines that need to be evaluated.

Greenish-white color:

Jaundice, or yellowing of the skin and eyes, along with nausea may indicate problems with the liver or gallbladder and need to be evaluated by a doctor right once.

Temperature spike:

When fever and nausea are present, it may indicate an inflammatory or infectious disease that has to be treated.

Persistent Nausea Associated with Pregnancy:

Hyperemesis gravidarum, or severe and persistent nausea in pregnancy, may necessitate medical attention in order to control symptoms and avoid dehydration.

Past Health Issues:

People who have experienced cancer, gastrointestinal issues, or liver disease in the past should be especially cautious about chronic nausea since it could indicate the advancement or return of their illness.

Drug-Related Problems:

Treatment modifications may be necessary if persistent nausea is a side effect of a medicine. When it comes to medication management, speaking with a healthcare professional is crucial.

It is imperative that you get urgent medical assistance if you experience chronic nausea along with any of these warning signs. An extensive assessment by a medical professional can assist in determining the underlying reason and directing the best course of action. This evaluation may involve a physical examination, lab testing, imaging studies, and other diagnostic procedures. Ignoring chronic nausea in the presence of warning signs could postpone the diagnosis and treatment of potentially dangerous illnesses.

Particular Populations' Nausea

Numerous unique demographics, such as distinct age groups and medical situations, are susceptible to nausea. When it comes to nausea in particular populations, keep the following in mind:

Individuals who are expecting (morning sickness):

During pregnancy, morning sickness is a frequent occurrence that usually happens in the first trimester. Although hyperemesis gravidarum, or severe or persistent nausea, usually poses minimal health risks to the mother or infant, it may necessitate medical attention in order to prevent dehydration and to give supportive care.

Kids:

A number of conditions, such as infections, motion sickness, gastrointestinal problems, or mental stress, can cause nausea in children. In order to treat the condition appropriately, the cause must be determined. If the nausea doesn't go away, parents should speak with a pediatrician.

Senior Citizens:

Nausea in older individuals might be brought on by age-related changes, adverse drug reactions, or underlying medical disorders. Healthcare professionals should attend to the unique requirements of older patients who are feeling nausea, as dehydration is a particular issue.

Individuals Receiving Chemotherapy:

One common side effect of chemotherapy is nausea. Antiemetic drugs are frequently administered to treat nausea and vomiting brought on by chemotherapy. For efficient symptom management, patients and their oncology team must communicate.

Individuals suffering from digestive disorders:

People who suffer from gastrointestinal illnesses including GERD, IBS, or IBD (irritable bowel disease) may have reflux disease (GERD) or endure chronic or recurrent nausea. The goal of treatment plans is to control the underlying gastrointestinal ailment.

Individuals with neurological conditions:

Nausea may be a symptom of some neurological illnesses, including brainstem problems, migraines, and vertigo. In order to manage the neurological disorder, supporting care must be given.

People Affected by Mental Health Issues:

Anxiety, sadness, and eating disorders are a few mental health issues that can manifest as nausea. Effective management requires addressing the underlying psychological causes and integrating mental health support.

People with Prolonged Illness:

Nausea is a common symptom of chronic conditions such as liver disease, renal disease, or autoimmune disorders. Important components of care include taking care of the underlying illness and meeting nutritional requirements.

Individuals Suffering from Drug-Induced Nausea:

Nausea is a side effect of various medications, such as opioids, chemotherapy treatments, and some antibiotics. It may be essential to add antiemetic drugs or modify prescription regimes.

Motion Sickness Sufferers:

People of all ages are susceptible to motion sickness, especially when traveling. Medication, acupressure, or gazing on the horizon to reduce motion-induced nausea are examples of preventive techniques.

It is crucial to modify the treatment of nausea in accordance with the unique requirements and traits of these particular groups. Developing a thorough management plan for nausea should take the patient's age, health, and underlying disorders into account.

CONCLUSION

In summary, nausea is a widespread and complicated symptom that can be brought on by a number of illnesses, drugs, psychological issues, and environmental cues. Periodic or acute nausea is usually a typical reaction to specific events, but persistent or severe nausea has to be treated by a doctor.

The key to managing nausea effectively is figuring out what the underlying cause is and treating it. A comprehensive medical history, physical examination, laboratory testing, imaging investigations, and consultation with medical specialists are all possible steps in the diagnosis process. Red flags should be evaluated by a doctor right away, such as sudden, unexplained weight loss, severe stomach pain, or dehydration symptoms.

A variety of techniques are used to treat nausea, such as pharmaceuticals, dietary adjustments, lifestyle adjustments, and psychological assistance. Comprehensive care requires that the treatment plan be customized to the patient's unique needs and that any related symptoms be addressed.

Considerations for managing nausea may differ in distinct populations, such as expectant mothers, young children, the elderly, and people with certain medical disorders. Specific strategies are needed for nausea brought on by chemotherapy, nausea connected to pregnancy, and nausea related to chronic conditions.

Relieving symptoms can be facilitated by coping mechanisms and lifestyle changes such as rest, acupressure, dietary changes, and increased hydration. However, in order to receive the proper evaluation and treatment, persistent or severe nausea should always be discussed with medical professionals.

Ultimately, the key to treating this symptom and enhancing the general wellbeing of those with nausea is to comprehend the underlying causes of the condition, incorporate appropriate remedies, and keep open contact with healthcare providers.

THE END